C000170828

The Vibrant Mediterranean Fish and Meat Recipe Collection

Amazing and Delicious Recipes for Incredible Meals and Eat Healthy

Camila Lester

Table of contents

Lime Chicken with Black Beans

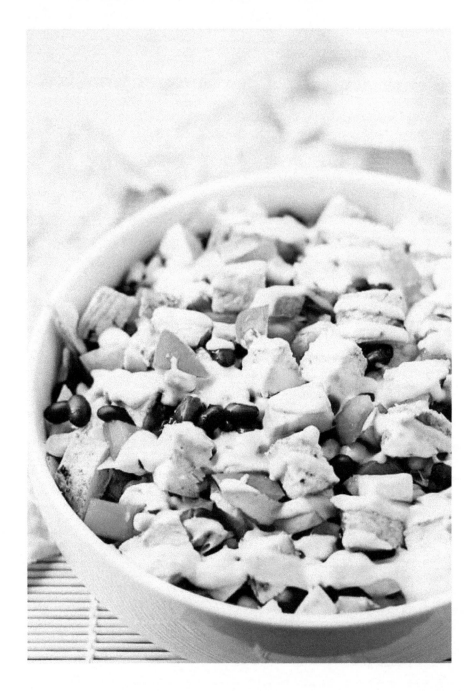

Difficulty Level: 2/5

Preparation time: 10 minutes

Cooking time: 10 minutes

Servings: 8

Ingredients:

8 chicken thighs (boneless and skinless)

3 tablespoons lime juice

1 cup black beans

1 cup canned tomatoes

4 teaspoons garlic powder

Directions:

Marinate the chicken in a mixture of lime juice and garlic powder.

Add the chicken to the Pressure Pot.

Pour the tomatoes on top of the chicken.

Seal the pot.

Set it to manual.

Cook at high pressure for 10 minutes.

Release the pressure naturally.

Stir in the black beans.

Press sauté to simmer until black beans are cooked.

Nutrition: (Per serving)

Calories 370

Total Fat 11.2g

Saturated Fat 3.1g

Cholesterol 130mg

Sodium 128mg

Total Carbohydrate 17.5g

Dietary Fiber 4.1g

Total Sugars 1.5g

Protein 47.9g

Potassium 790mg

Turkey Verde with Brown Rice
Difficulty Level: 2/5

Preparation time: 5 minutes

Cooking time: 25

Servings: 5

Ingredients:

2/3 cup chicken broth

1 1/4 cup brown rice

1 1/2 lb. turkey tenderloins

1 onion, sliced

1/2 cup salsa verde

Directions:

Add the chicken broth and rice to the Pressure Pot.

Top with the turkey, onion and salsa.

Cover the pot.

Set it to manual.

Cook at high pressure for 18 minutes.

Release the pressure naturally.

Wait for 8 minutes before opening the pot.

Nutrition: (Per serving)

Calories 336

Total Fat 3.3g

Saturated Fat 0.3g

Cholesterol 54mg

Sodium 321mg

Total Carbohydrate 39.4g

Dietary Fiber 2.2g

Total Sugars 1.4g

Protein 38.5g

Potassium 187mg

Turkey with Basil & Tomatoes
Difficulty Level: 2/5

Preparation time: 5 minutes

Cooking time: 10 minutes

Serves: 4

Ingredients:

4 turkey breast fillets

1 tablespoon olive oil

1/4 cup fresh basil, chopped

1 1/2 cups cherry tomatoes, sliced in half

1/4 cup olive tapenade

Directions:

Season the turkey fillets with salt.

Add the olive oil to the Pressure Pot.

Set it to sauté.

Cook the turkey until brown on both sides.

Stir in the basil, tomatoes and olive tapenade.

Cook for 3 minutes, stirring frequently.

Nutrition: (Per serving)

Calories 188

Total Fat 5.1g

Saturated Fat 1g

Cholesterol 0mg

Sodium 3mg

Total Carbohydrate 2.8g

Dietary Fiber 1.6g

Total Sugars 1.9g

Protein 33.2g

Potassium 164mg

Turkey Lasagna
Difficulty Level: 2/5

Preparation time: 20 minutes

Cooking time: 10 minutes

Servings: 4

Ingredients:

4 tortillas

1 1/4 cup salsa

1/2 can refried beans

1 1/2 cups cooked turkey

1 1/4 cup cheddar cheese, shredded

Directions:

Spray a small pan with oil.

Spread the refried beans on each tortilla.

Place the first tortilla inside the pan.

Add layers of the turkey, salsa and cheese.

Place another tortilla and repeat the layers.

Pour 1 cup of water inside the Pressure Pot.

Place the layers on top of a steamer basket.

Place the basket inside the Pressure Pot.

Choose manual setting.

Cook at high pressure for 10 minutes.

Nutrition: (Per serving)

Calories 335

Total Fat 15.5g

Saturated Fat 8.6g

Cholesterol 79mg

Sodium 849mg

Total Carbohydrate 21.1g

Dietary Fiber 4.5g

Total Sugars 3g

Protein 28.5g

Potassium 561mg

Tuna with Lemon Butter Sauce

Difficulty Level: 2/5

Preparation time: 10 minutes

Cooking time: 5 minutes

Servings: 4

Ingredients:

4 tuna fillets

1/4 cup lemon juice

1 tablespoon fresh dill

1 tablespoon butter

Directions:

Pour 1 cup water and lemon juice in the Pressure Pot.

Add the steamer basket.

Put the tuna fillet on top of the basket.

Season with salt and pepper and dill.

Seal the pot.

Choose manual setting.

Cook at high pressure for 5 minutes.

Release the pressure quickly.

Remove from the pot.

Place the butter on top.

Let it melt and then serve.

Nutrition: (Per serving)

Calories 213

Total Fat 18.5g

Saturated Fat 1.9g

Cholesterol 8mg

Sodium 25mg

Total Carbohydrate 0.8g

Dietary Fiber 0.2g

Total Sugars 0.3g

Protein 10.8g

Potassium 46mg

Mediterranean Cod

Difficulty Level: 2/5

Preparation time: 10 minutes

Cooking time: 10 minutes

Servings: 6

Ingredients:

6 cod fillets

1 onion, sliced

1 tablespoon lemon juice

1 teaspoon oregano

28 oz. canned diced tomatoes

Directions:

Season the cod with salt and pepper.

Add 2 tablespoons olive oil into the Pressure Pot.

Set it to sauté.

Add the cod and cook for 3 minutes per side.

Add the rest of the ingredients. Mix well.

Cover the pot.

Choose manual function.

Cook at high pressure for 5 minutes.

Release the pressure quickly.

Pour the sauce over the cod before serving.

Nutrition: (Per serving)

Calories 123

Total Fat 1.3g

Saturated Fat 0.1g

Cholesterol 55mg

Sodium 78mg

Total Carbohydrate 7.1g

Dietary Fiber 2.1g

Total Sugars 4.3g

Protein 21.4g

Potassium 348mg

Shrimp with Tomatoes & Feta

Difficulty Level: 2/5

Preparation time: 10 minutes

Cooking time: 10 minutes

Servings: 4

Ingredients:

2 tablespoons butter

1 tablespoon garlic, minced

1 lb. shrimp, peeled and deveined

14 oz. canned crushed tomatoes

1 cup feta cheese, crumbled

Directions:

Set the Pressure Pot to sauté.

Add the butter.

Wait for it to melt.

Add the garlic and cook until fragrant.

Add the shrimp and tomatoes.

Seal the pot.

Set it to manual.

Cook at low pressure for 1 minute.

Release the pressure quickly.

Top with the feta cheese.

Nutrition: (Per serving)

Calories 218

Total Fat 10.5g

Saturated Fat 6.6g

Cholesterol 192mg

Sodium 618mg

Total Carbohydrate 7.9g

Dietary Fiber 2.2g

Total Sugars 4.7g

Protein 22.5g

Potassium 150mg

Mussels in Garlic Butter Sauce

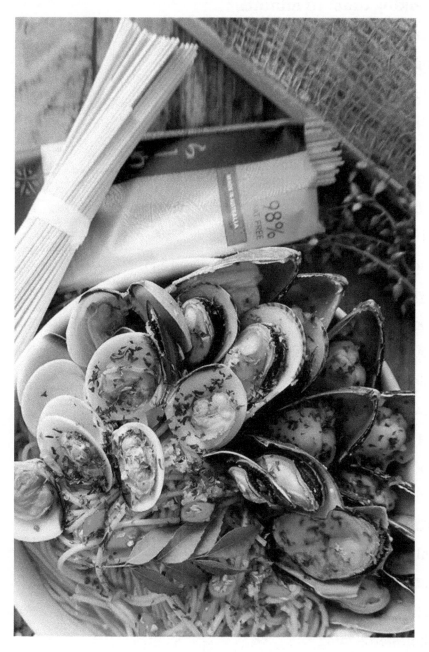

Difficulty Level: 2/5

Preparation time: 10 minutes

Cooking time: 10 minutes

Servings: 4

Ingredients:

2 tablespoons butter

4 cloves garlic, minced

1/2 cup broth

1/2 cup white wine

2 lb. mussels, cleaned and beard removed

Directions:

Add the butter and garlic in the Pressure Pot.

Switch it to sauté.

Cook until fragrant.

Pour in the broth and wine.

Add the mussels.

Cover the pot.

Set it to manual.

Cook at high pressure for 5 minutes.

Release the pressure quickly.

Nutrition: (Per serving)

Calories 280

Total Fat 11g

Saturated Fat 4.7g

Cholesterol 79mg

Sodium 787mg

Total Carbohydrate 10.3g

Dietary Fiber 0.1g

Total Sugars 0.4g

Protein 27.9g

Potassium 795mg

Fish Stew with Tomatoes & Olives

Difficulty Level: 2/5

Preparation time: 5 minutes

Cooking time: 10 minutes

Servings: 4

Ingredients:

1 1/2 lb. halibut fillet

4 cloves garlic, minced

1 cup cherry tomatoes, sliced in half

3 cups tomato soup

1 cup green olives, pitted and sliced

Directions:

Season the fish with salt and pepper.

Pour 1 tablespoon olive oil into the Pressure Pot.

Add the garlic and cook until fragrant.

Add the fish.

Cook for 3 minutes per side.

Add the rest of the ingredients.

Cover the pot.

Select manual function.

Cook at low pressure for 3 minutes.

Release the pressure quickly.

Nutrition: (Per serving)

Calories 245

Total Fat 3.7g

Saturated Fat 0.6g

Cholesterol 35mg

Sodium 1098mg

Total Carbohydrate 28g

Dietary Fiber 2.9g

Total Sugars 16.5g

Protein 26.3g

Potassium 1040mg

Rosemary Salmon
Difficulty Level: 2/5

Preparation time: 10 minutes

Cooking time: 5 minutes

Servings: 3

Ingredients:

1 lb. salmon fillets

10 oz. fresh asparagus

1 sprig fresh rosemary

1/2 cup cherry tomatoes, sliced in half

Dressing (mixture of 1 tablespoon olive oil and 1 tablespoon lemon juice)

Directions:

Add 1 cup of water into the Pressure Pot.

Place the steamer rack inside.

Put the salmon fillets on the rack.

Add the rosemary and asparagus on top of the salmon.

Cover the pot.

Select manual setting.

Cook at high pressure for 3 minutes.

Release the pressure quickly.

Transfer to a plate.

Place the tomatoes on the side.

Drizzle with the dressing.

Nutrition: (Per serving)

Calories 267

Total Fat 14.3g

Saturated Fat 2.1g

Cholesterol 67mg

Sodium 71mg

Total Carbohydrate 5.2g

Dietary Fiber 2.5g

Total Sugars 2.7g

Protein 31.7g

Potassium 853mg

Salmon with Tahini Sauce
Difficulty Level: 2/5

Preparation time: 5 minutes

Cooking time: 5 minutes

Servings: 2

Ingredients:

1 lb. salmon fillets

3 tablespoons tahini sauce

2 lemon slices

2 sprigs fresh rosemary

Directions:

Add the water to the Pressure Pot.

Place a steamer basket inside.

Put the salmon on top of the basket.

Season with salt and pepper.

Place rosemary and lemon slice on top.

Cover the pot.

Set it to manual.

Cook at high pressure for 3 minutes.

Release the pressure quickly.

Drizzle the tahini sauce on top before serving.

Nutrition: (Per serving)

Calories 306

Total Fat 14.2g

Saturated Fat 2.1g

Cholesterol 100mg

Sodium 101mg

Total Carbohydrate 1.4g

Dietary Fiber 0.7g

Total Sugars 0.2g

Protein 44.1g

Potassium 892mg

Fish & Potatoes
Difficulty Level: 2/5

Preparation time: 5 minutes

Cooking time: 10 minutes

Servings: 4

Ingredients:

1 lb. cod fillets, sliced into strips.

1 onion, chopped

1 lb. potatoes, sliced into cubes

4 cups vegetable broth

1 teaspoon old bay seasoning

Directions:

Season the salmon fillets with salt and pepper.

Pour 1 tablespoon olive oil in the Pressure Pot.

Add the onion.

Cook for 3 minutes.

Add the salmon and cook for 1 minute per side.

Pour in the broth and add the potatoes and seasoning.

Seal the pot.

Turn it to manual.

Cook at high pressure for 3 minutes.

Release the pressure quickly.

Nutrition: (Per serving)

Calories 278

Total Fat 8.5g

Saturated Fat 1.4g

Cholesterol 50mg

Sodium 981mg

Total Carbohydrate 21.3g

Dietary Fiber 3.3g

Total Sugars 3.2g

Protein 29.1g

Potassium 1144mg

Sautéed Shrimp with Garlic Couscous
Difficulty Level: 2/5

Preparation time: 5 minutes

Cooking time: 5 minutes

Servings: 4

Ingredients:

1 lb. shrimp, peeled and deveined

1/2 cup fresh chives, chopped

1/2 cup fresh parsley, chopped

1 tablespoon scallions, chopped

10 oz. garlic flavored couscous

Directions:

Choose sauté function in the Pressure Pot.

Add 2 tablespoons of olive oil.

Add the shrimp and herbs.

Cook for 3 minutes, stirring frequently.

Serve with the couscous.

Nutrition: (Per serving)

Calories 615

Total Fat 8.3g

Saturated Fat 0.6g

Cholesterol 239mg

Sodium 1556mg

Total Carbohydrate 95g

Dietary Fiber 8g

Total Sugars 2.7g

Protein 43.8g

Potassium 256mg

Salmon with Garlic & Basil Potatoes

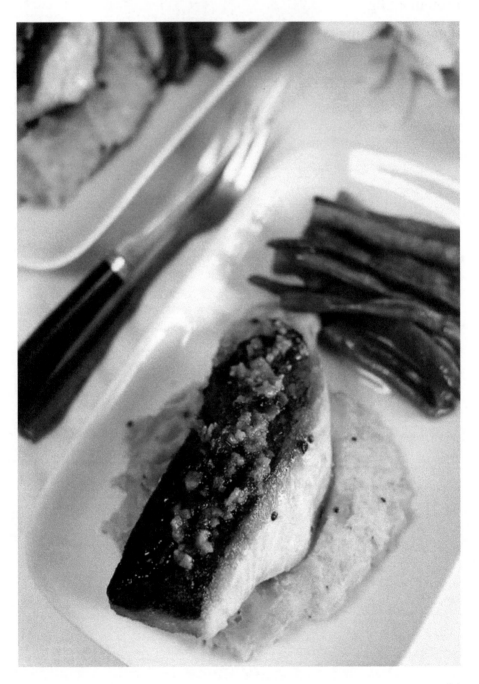

Difficulty Level: 2/5

Preparation time: 5 minutes

Cooking time: 5 minutes

Servings: 4

Ingredients:

1 lb. baby potatoes

4 tablespoons butter, divided

4 salmon fillets

4 cloves garlic, minced

1 teaspoon dried basil

Directions:

Put the potatoes in the Pressure Pot.

Add 1 cup water and half of the butter.

Season with salt and pepper.

Put the steamer rack inside the pot, over the potatoes.

Sprinkle both sides of salmon with salt and pepper.

Seal the pot and set it to manual. Cook at high pressure for 3 minutes.

Transfer the salmon to a plate.

Remove the potatoes and slice each in half.

Add the remaining butter to the pot.

Add the garlic and cook until fragrant.

Put the potatoes back to the pot.

Sprinkle with basil leaves.

Cook for 1 minute.

Serve salmon with potatoes.

Nutrition: (Per serving)

Calories 408

Total Fat 22.6g

Saturated Fat 8.9g

Cholesterol 109mg

Sodium 172mg

Total Carbohydrate 15.1g

Dietary Fiber 2.9g

Total Sugars 0g

Protein 37.8g

Potassium 1168mg

Sauce Dipped Mussels
Difficulty Level: 2/5

Preparation Time: 20 minutes

Cooking time: 10 minutes

Servings: 4

Ingredients:

2 green chilies, deseeded and chopped

2 shallots, finely diced

4 tablespoons olive oil

4 ripe tomatoes, soaked, drained and diced

2 garlic cloves, minced

2 glasses dry white wine

2 handfuls basil leaves

2 pounds mussels, cleaned

2 pinches sugar

2 teaspoons tomato paste

Salt and black pepper, to taste

Directions:

Heat olive oil in a skillet and stir in garlic, green chilies and shallots.

Sauté for about 3 minutes and add salt, black pepper, sugar, wine and tomatoes.

Cook for about 2 minutes and add mussels.

Cover with a lid and cook for about 5 minutes.

Garnish with basil leaves and immediately serve.

Nutrition:

Calories 320

Total Fat 17.8 g

Saturated Fat 2.7 g

Cholesterol 42 mg

Total Carbs 19.4 g

Dietary Fiber 2.4 g

Sugar 6.8 g

Protein 20.3 g

Mixed Seafood Stew

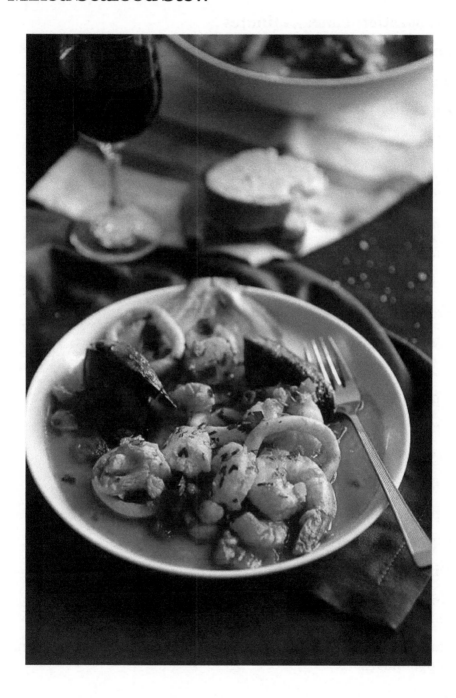

Difficulty Level: 2/5

Preparation Time: 5 minutes

Cooking time: 25 minutes

Servings: 8

Ingredients:

2 tablespoons olive oil

2 teaspoons lemon peel, grated

2/3 cup white wine

2 medium onions, finely chopped

3 teaspoons garlic, minced and divided

1-pound plum tomatoes, seeded and diced

½ teaspoon red pepper flakes, crushed

2 tablespoons tomato paste

2 oz. red snapper fillets, cut into 1-inch cubes

2 pounds shrimps, peeled and deveined

2 cups clam juice

2/3 cup mayonnaise, reduced-fat

Salt, to taste

1-pound sea scallops

2/3 cup fresh parsley, minced

Directions:

Heat olive oil in a Dutch oven on medium heat and add garlic and onions.

Sauté for about 3 minutes and add tomatoes, lemon peel and pepper flakes.

Sauté for about 2 minutes and stir in wine, salt, tomato paste and clam juice.

Boil this mixture and reduce it to a simmer.

Cover the lid and cook for about 10 minutes.

Toss in the shrimps, scallops, parsley and red snapper fillets.

Cover and cook for 10 more minutes and serve topped with garlic and mayonnaise.

Nutrition:

Calories 390

Total Fat 15.3 g

Saturated Fat 2.6 g

Cholesterol 261 mg

Total Carbs 20.1 g

Dietary Fiber 1.9 g

Sugar 7.3 g

Protein 39 g

Seafood Garlic Couscous
Difficulty Level: 2/5

Preparation Time: 10 minutes

Cooking time: 20 minutes

Servings: 8

Ingredients:

8 scallions, sliced

4 (5.4-oz.) boxes garlic-flavored couscous, boiled and drained

1-pound raw shrimp, peeled, deveined and coarsely chopped

1 cup fresh parsley, chopped

4 tablespoons olive oil

2 pounds codfish, cut into 1-inch pieces

1 cup fresh chives, chopped

Hot sauce, to taste

1-pound bay scallops

Salt and black pepper, to taste

Directions:

Mix shrimps, scallions, codfish, scallops, parsley, chives, salt and black pepper in a bowl.

Heat oil in a deep skillet and add the seafood mixture.

Sauté until golden and pour in the hot sauce.

Lower the heat and cover with a lid.

Divide the couscous into the serving plates and top evenly with the seafood mixture.

Dish out and serve immediately.

Nutrition:

Calories 476

Total Fat 9 g

Saturated Fat 1.4 g

Cholesterol 138 mg

Total Carbs 68 g

Dietary Fiber 4.9 g

Sugar 0.8 g

Protein 32.9 g

Crusty Grilled Clams
Difficulty Level: 2/5

Preparation Time: 5 minutes

Cooking time: 10 minutes

Servings: 4

Ingredients:

4 tablespoons garlic and parsley butter

2 cups toasted bread crumbs

Fresh herbs, to garnish

2 pounds clams, rinsed and debearded

Chopped tomatoes, to garnish

2 lemons, zested

Directions:

Boil clams in a water for about 3 minutes in a large pot.

Preheat the grill and lightly grease a baking sheet.

Mix zest and bread crumbs in a bowl.

Drizzle butter on top of the clams and place them shell side down on the baking sheet.

Top the bread crumbs mixture on the clams and transfer to the grill.

Cover the grill for about 4 minutes and let it cook.

Serve garnished with tomato and parsley.

Nutrition:

Calories 510

Total Fat 19.5 g

Saturated Fat 8.9 g

Cholesterol 94 mg

Total Carbs 47.3 g

Dietary Fiber 2.4 g

Sugar 3.4 g

Protein 34.3 g

Lemon-Thyme Chicken

Difficulty Level: 2/5

Preparation Time: 5 minutes

Cooking time: 25 minutes

Servings: 8

Ingredients:

½ teaspoon black pepper

2 teaspoons crushed dried thyme, divided

8 small skinless, boneless chicken breast halves

2 lemons, thinly sliced

1 teaspoon salt

4 garlic cloves, minced

8 teaspoons extra-virgin olive oil, divided

2 pounds fingerling potatoes, halved lengthwise

Directions:

Heat half of olive oil in a skillet over medium heat and add ½ teaspoon thyme, potatoes, salt and black pepper.

Cover and cook for about 12 minutes, while stirring occasionally.

Push the potatoes to a side and add rest of the olive oil and chicken.

Sear the chicken for about 5 minutes per side and season with thyme.

Arrange lemon slices over the chicken and cover the pan.

Cook for about 10 minutes and dish out to serve hot.

Nutrition:

Calories 483

Total Fat 9.4 g

Saturated Fat 0.7 g

Cholesterol 195 mg

Total Carbs 18.8 g

Dietary Fiber 2.1 g

Sugar 1.2 g

Protein 80.3 g

Mediterranean Chicken Quinoa Bowl

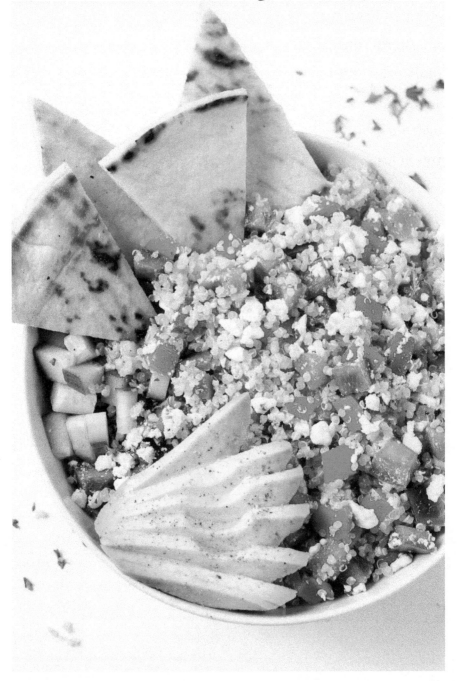

Difficulty Level: 2/5

Preparation Time: 10 minutes

Cooking time: 15 minutes

Servings: 8

Ingredients:

½ cup almonds, slivered

1/8 teaspoon black pepper

2 tablespoons extra-virgin olive oil, divided

1/8 teaspoon crushed red pepper

1 tablespoon fresh parsley, finely chopped

1 cup cooked quinoa

1/8 cup feta cheese, crumbled

½ teaspoon salt

1 small garlic clove, crushed

½ pound boneless, skinless chicken breasts, trimmed

½ (7-ounce) jar roasted red peppers, rinsed

½ teaspoon paprika

1/8 cup pitted Kalamata olives, chopped

½ cup cucumber, diced

¼ teaspoon ground cumin

1/8 cup red onions, finely chopped

Directions:

Preheat the oven on broiler setting and lightly grease a baking sheet.

Sprinkle the chicken with salt and black pepper.

Transfer it on the baking sheet and broil for about 15 minutes.

Let the chicken cool for about 5 minutes and transfer to a cutting board.

Shred the chicken and keep aside.

Put almonds, paprika, black pepper, garlic, half of olive oil, red pepper and cumin in a blender.

Blend until smooth and dish out in a bowl.

Toss quinoa, red onions, 2 tablespoons oil, quinoa and olives in a bowl.

Divide the quinoa mixture in the serving bowls and top with cucumber, red pepper sauce and chicken.

Garnish with feta cheese and parsley to immediately serve.

Nutrition:

Calories 741

Total Fat 33.7 g

Saturated Fat 6.7 g

Cholesterol 109 mg

Total Carbs 62.1 g

Dietary Fiber 8.2 g

Sugar 3.6 g

Protein 48.4 g

Blue Cheese-Topped Pork Chops
Difficulty Level: 2/5

Preparation Time: 10 minutes

Cooking time: 15 minutes

Servings: 8

Ingredients:

4 tablespoons fat-free Italian salad dressing

½ cup reduced-fat blue cheese, crumbled

2 pinches cayenne pepper

8 (6-ounce) bone-in pork loin chops

2 tablespoons fresh rosemary, snipped

Directions:

Preheat the oven at broiler settings and line a broiler tray with a foil sheet.

Mix the Italian salad dressing with cayenne pepper.

Brush the dressing mixture on both sides of the pork chops.

Place the pork chops on the broiler tray and broil the pork chops for about 10 minutes, flipping in between.

Top the chops with blue cheese and rosemary to serve.

Nutrition:

Calories 506

Total Fat 21.6 g

Saturated Fat 3.7 g

Cholesterol 193 mg

Total Carbs 3.3 g

Dietary Fiber 0.9 g

Sugar 1.6 g

Protein 70.8 g

Greek Beef Steak and Hummus Plate

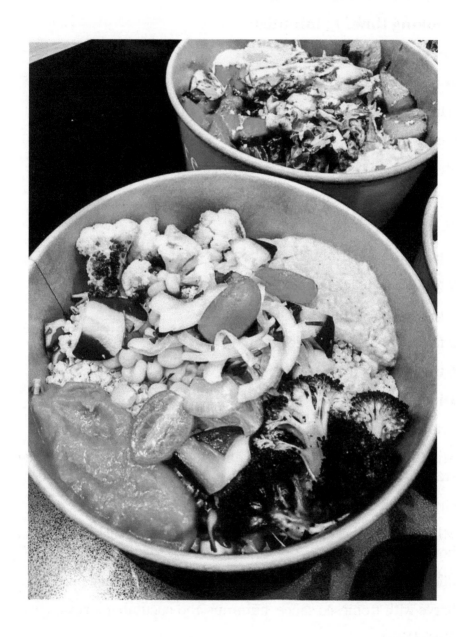

Difficulty Level: 2/5

Preparation Time: 10 minutes

Cooking time: 15 minutes

Servings: 8

Ingredients:

2 tablespoons plus 2 teaspoons garlic, minced

2 cups hummus

½ cup fresh oregano leaves, chopped

2 medium cucumbers, thinly sliced

½ teaspoon black pepper

2 pounds beef sirloin steaks, boneless, cut 1 inch thick

2 teaspoons black pepper

4 tablespoons Romesco Sauce

2 tablespoons lemon peel, grated

6 tablespoons fresh lemon juice

Directions:

Preheat a grill on medium heat and lightly grease a grill grate.

Mix together all the dry spices and rub on both sides of the beef steaks.

Grill the steaks for about 15 minutes.

Mix together sliced cucumber, lemon juice and black pepper in a bowl.

Slice the grilled steak and sprinkle with salt and black pepper.

Serve with Romesco sauce, hummus and cucumber strips.

Nutrition:

Calories 463

Total Fat 37.7 g

Saturated Fat 7.6 g

Cholesterol 28 mg

Total Carbs 68.7 g

Dietary Fiber 14.5 g

Sugar 19.7 g

Protein 36.4 g

Linguine with Shrimp
Difficulty Level: 2/5

Preparation time: 10 minutes

Cooking time: 15 minutes

Servings: 4

Ingredients:

3 tablespoons extra virgin olive oil

12 ounces linguine

1 tablespoon garlic, minced

30 large shrimp, peeled and deveined

A pinch of red pepper flakes, crushed

1 cup green olives, pitted and chopped

3 tablespoons lemon juice

1 teaspoon lemon zest, grated

¼ cup parsley, chopped

Directions:

Put some water in a large saucepan, add water, bring to a boil over medium high heat, add linguine, cook according to instructions, take off heat, drain and put in a bowl and reserve ½ cup cooking liquid.

Heat a pan with 2 tablespoons oil over medium high heat, add shrimp, stir and cook for 3 minutes.

Add pepper flakes and garlic, stir and cook 10 seconds more.

Add remaining oil, lemon zest and juice and stir well.

Add pasta and olives, reserved cooking liquid and parsley, stir, cook for 2 minutes more, take off heat, divide between plates and serve.

Nutrition:

Calories 500,

Fat 20,

Fiber 5,

Carbs 45,

Protein 34

Oysters with Vinaigrette

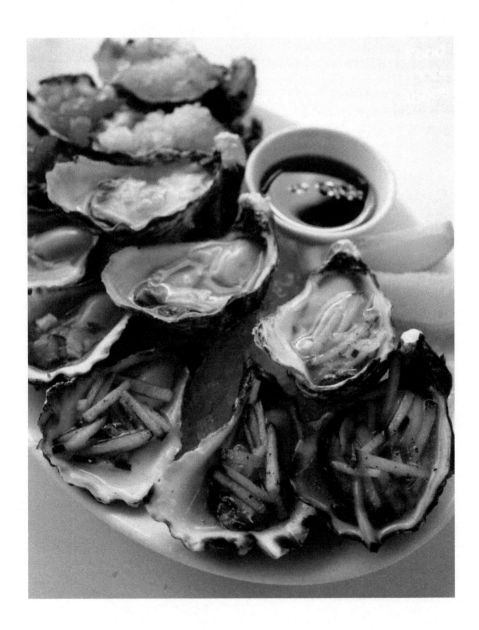

Difficulty Level: 2/5

Preparation time: 10 minutes

Cooking time: 6 minutes

Servings: 4

Ingredients:

2 tablespoons shallots, finely chopped

½ cup sherry vinegar

A pinch of saffron threads

½ cup olive oil

1 tablespoon olive oil

Salt and black pepper to taste

1 pound chorizo sausage, chopped

1 pound fennel bulbs, thinly sliced lengthwise

24 oysters, shucked

Directions:

In a bowl, mix shallots with vinegar, saffron, salt, pepper and ½ cup olive oil and stir well.

Heat a pan with the remaining oil over medium high heat, add sausage, cook for 4 minutes, transfer to a paper towel, drain grease and put on a plate.

Add fennel on top, spoon vinaigrette into each oyster and place them on the platter as well, drizzle the rest of the vinaigrette on top and serve.

Nutrition:

Calories 113,

Fat 1,

Fiber 3,
Carbs 10,
Protein 7

Shrimp with Honeydew and Feta

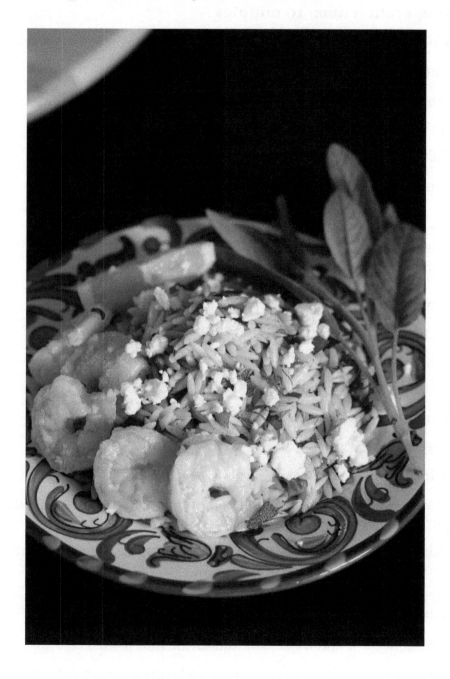

Difficulty Level: 2/5

Preparation time: 10 minutes

Cooking time: 4 minutes

Servings: 4

Ingredients:

30 big shrimp, peeled and deveined

Salt and black pepper to taste

A pinch of cayenne pepper

¼ cup olive oil

2 tablespoons shallots, chopped

1 teaspoon lime zest

4 teaspoons lime juice

½ pound frisee or curly endive, torn into small pieces

1 honeydew melon, peeled, seeded and chopped

¼ cup mint, chopped

8 ounces feta cheese, crumbled

1 tablespoon coriander seeds

Directions:

Heat a pan with 2 tablespoons oil over medium high heat, add shrimp, cook for 1 minute and flip.

Add lime zest, 1 teaspoon lime juice, shallots and some salt, stir, cook for 1 minute and take off heat.

In a bowl, mix the remaining oil with the rest of the lime juice, salt and pepper to taste.

Add honeydew and frisee, stir and divide into plates.

Add shrimp, coriander seeds, mint and feta on top and serve.

Nutrition:

Calories 245,

Fat 23,

Fiber 3,

Carbs 23,

Protein 45

Spicy Seared Mussels
Difficulty Level: 2/5

Preparation time: 10 minutes

Cooking time: 15 minutes

Servings: 4

Ingredients:

1 and ½ cups green grapes, cut in quarters

Zest from 1 lemon, chopped

Juice of 1 lemon

Salt and black pepper to taste

2 scallions, chopped

¼ cup olive oil

2 tablespoons mint, chopped

2 tablespoons cilantro, chopped

1 teaspoon cumin, ground

1 teaspoon paprika

½ teaspoon ginger, ground

¼ teaspoon cinnamon, ground

1 teaspoon turmeric, ground

½ cup water

1 and ½ pounds sea scallops

Directions:

Heat a pan with the water, some salt and the lemon zest over medium high heat and simmer for 10 minutes.

Drain lemon zest and transfer to a bowl.

Mix with grapes, 2 tablespoons oil, cilantro, mint and scallions and stir well.

In another bowl, mix cumin with turmeric, paprika, cinnamon and ginger and stir.

Season scallops with salt and pepper, coat with the spice mix and place them on a plate.

Heat a pan with remaining oil over medium high heat, add scallops, cook for 2 minutes on each side and transfer to a plate.

Divide scallops on 4 plates, pour lemon juice over them and serve with grape relish.

Nutrition:

Calories 320,

Fat 12,

Fiber 2,

Carbs 18,

Protein 28

Shrimps with Lemon and Pepper

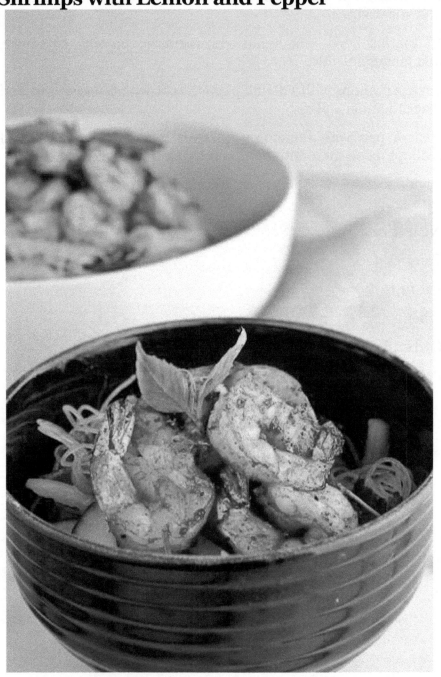

Difficulty Level: 2/5

Preparation time: 10 minutes

Cooking time: 3 minutes

Servings: 4

Ingredients:

40 big shrimp, peeled and deveined

6 garlic cloves, minced

Salt and black pepper to taste

3 tablespoons olive oil

¼ teaspoon sweet paprika

A pinch of red pepper flakes, crushed

¼ teaspoon lemon zest, grated

3 tablespoons sherry

1 and ½ tablespoons chives, sliced

Juice of 1 lemon

Directions:

Heat a pan with the oil over medium high heat, add shrimp, season with salt and pepper and cook for 1 minute.

Add paprika, garlic and pepper flakes, stir and cook for 1 minute.

Add sherry, stir and cook for 1 minute more.

Take shrimp off heat, add chives and lemon zest, stir and transfer shrimp to plates. Add lemon juice all over and serve.

Nutrition:

Calories 140,

Fat 1,

Fiber 0,

Carbs 1,

Protein 18

Zucchini and Chicken

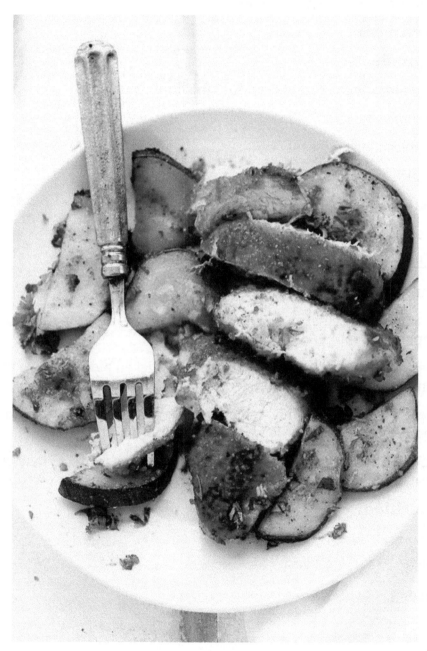

Difficulty Level: 2/5

Preparation time: 10 minutes

Cooking time: 15 minutes

Servings: 4

Ingredients:

1 pound chicken breasts, cut into medium chunks

12 ounces zucchini, sliced

2 tablespoons olive oil

2 garlic cloves, minced

2 tablespoons parmesan, grated

1 tablespoon parsley, chopped

Salt and black pepper to taste

Directions:

In a bowl, mix chicken pieces with 1 tablespoon oil, some salt and pepper and toss to coat.

Heat a pan over medium high heat, add chicken pieces, brown for 6 minutes on all sides, transfer to a plate and leave aside.

Heat the pan with the remaining oil over medium heat, add zucchini slices and garlic, stir and cook for 5 minutes.

Return chicken pieces to pan, add parmesan on top, stir, take off heat, divide between plates and serve with some parsley on top.

Nutrition:

Calories 212,

Fat 4,

Fiber 3,

Carbs 4,

Protein 7

Grilled Chicken Wraps
Difficulty Level: 2/5

Preparation time: 10 minutes

Cooking time: 12 minutes

Servings: 4

Ingredients:

4 chicken breast halves, skinless and boneless

Salt and black pepper to taste

4 teaspoons olive oil

1 small cucumber, sliced

3 teaspoons cilantro, chopped

4 Greek whole wheat tortillas

4 tablespoons peanut sauce

Directions:

Heat a grill pan over medium high heat, season chicken with salt and pepper, rub with the oil, add to the grill, cook for 6 minutes on each side, transfer to a cutting board, leave to cool down for 5 minutes, slice and leave aside.

In a bowl, mix cilantro with cucumber and stir.

Heat a pan over medium heat, add each tortilla, heat up for 20 seconds and transfer them to a working surface.

Spread 1 tablespoon peanut sauce on each tortilla, divide chicken and cucumber mix on each, fold, arrange on plates and serve.

Nutrition:

Calories 321,

Fat 3,

Fiber 4,

Carbs 7,
Protein 9

Pork Chops and Relish

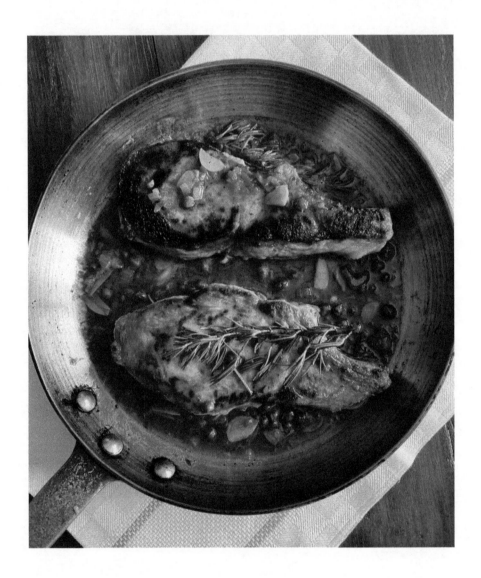

Difficulty Level: 2/5

Preparation time: 15 minutes

Cooking time: 14 minutes

Servings: 6

Ingredients:

6 pork chops, boneless

7 ounces marinated artichoke hearts, chopped and their liquid reserved

A pinch of salt and black pepper

1 teaspoon hot pepper sauce

1 and ½ cups tomatoes, cubed

1 jalapeno pepper, chopped

½ cup roasted bell peppers, chopped

½ cup black olives, pitted and sliced

Directions:

In a bowl, mix the chops with the pepper sauce, reserved liquid from the artichokes, cover and keep in the fridge for 15 minutes.

Heat up a grill over medium-high heat, add the pork chops and cook for 7 minutes on each side.

In a bowl, combine the artichokes with the peppers and the remaining ingredients, toss, divide on top of the chops and serve.

Nutrition:

Calories 215,

Fat 6,

Fiber 1,

Carbs 6,

Protein 35

Glazed Pork Chops
Difficulty Level: 2/5

Preparation time: 10 minutes

Cooking time: 20 minutes

Servings: 4

Ingredients:

¼ cup apricot preserves

4 pork chops, boneless

1 tablespoon thyme, chopped

½ teaspoon cinnamon powder

2 tablespoons olive oil

Directions:

Heat up a pan with the oil over medium-high heat, add the apricot preserves and cinnamon, whisk, bring to a simmer, cook for 10 minutes and take off the heat.

Heat up your grill over medium-high heat, brush the pork chops with some of the apricot glaze, place them on the grill and cook for 10 minutes.

Flip the chops, brush them with more apricot glaze, cook for 10 minutes more and divide between plates.

Sprinkle the thyme on top and serve.

Nutrition:

Calories 225,

Fat 11,

Fiber 0,

Carbs 6,

Protein 23

Pork Chops and Cherries Mix
Difficulty Level: 2/5

Preparation time: 10 minutes

Cooking time: 12 minutes

Servings: 4

Ingredients:

4 pork chops, boneless

Salt and black pepper to the taste

½ cup cranberry juice

1 and ½ teaspoons spicy mustard

½ cup dark cherries, pitted and halved

Cooking spray

Directions:

Heat up a pan greased with the cooking spray over medium-high heat, add the pork chops, cook them for 5 minutes on each side and divide between plates.

Heat up the same pan over medium heat, add the cranberry juice and the rest of the ingredients, whisk, bring to a simmer, cook for 2 minutes, drizzle over the pork chops and serve.

Nutrition:

Calories 262,

Fat 8,

Fiber 1,

Carbs 16,

Protein 30

Pork Chops and Herbed Tomato Sauce
Difficulty Level: 2/5

Preparation time: 10 minutes

Cooking time: 10 minutes

Servings: 4

Ingredients:

4 pork loin chops, boneless

6 tomatoes, peeled and crushed

3 tablespoons parsley, chopped

2 tablespoons olive oil

¼ cup kalamata olives, pitted and halved

1 yellow onion, chopped

1 garlic clove, minced

Directions:

Heat up a pan with the oil over medium heat, add the pork chops, cook them for 3 minutes on each side and divide between plates.

Heat up the same pan again over medium heat, add the tomatoes, parsley and the rest of the ingredients, whisk, simmer for 4 minutes, drizzle over the chops and serve.

Nutrition:

Calories 334,

Fat 17,

Fiber 2,

Carbs 12,

Protein 34

Black Bean & Turkey Skillet

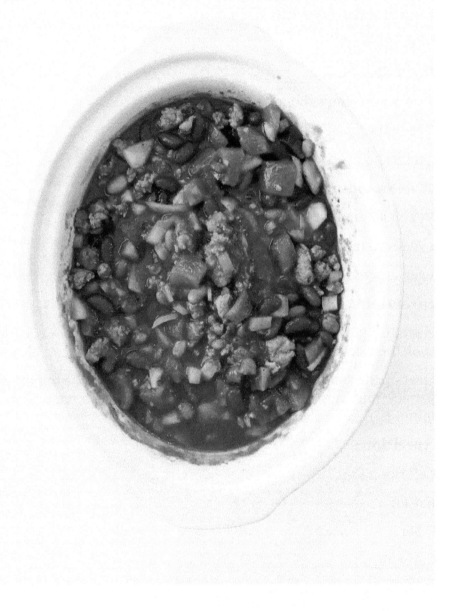

Difficulty Level: 2/5

Preparation time: 20 minutes

Cooking time: 10 mins

Servings: 6

Ingredients

1 tablespoon olive oil

20 oz. lean ground turkey

2 medium zucchinis, cut into slices

1 medium onion, chopped

2 banana peppers, seeded and chopped

3 garlic cloves, minced

1/2 teaspoon dried oregano

1 x 15 oz. can black beans, rinsed and drained

1 x 14.5 oz. can diced tomatoes, undrained

1 tablespoon balsamic vinegar

1/2 teaspoon salt

Directions:

Grab a large skillet, add the oil and pop over a medium heat.

Add the turkey, zucchini, onion, peppers, garlic and oregano and cook for 10 minutes.

Stir through the remaining ingredients and cook long enough to heat through then serve and enjoy.

Nutrition: (Per serving)

Calories: 259

Net carbs: 6g

Fat: 10g

Protein: 24g

Beef Kofta
Difficulty Level: 2/5

Preparation time: 10 minutes

Cooking time: 15 mins

Servings: 4

Ingredients

1 lb. ground beef

1/2 cup minced onions

1 tablespoon olive oil

1/2 teaspoon salt

1/2 teaspoon ground coriander

1/2 teaspoon ground cumin

1/4 teaspoon ground cinnamon

1/4 teaspoon allspice

1/4 teaspoon dried mint leaves

Directions:

Grab a large bowl and add all the ingredients.

Stir well to combine then use your hands to shape into ovals or balls.

Carefully thread onto skewers then brush with oil.

Pop into the grill and cook uncovered for 15 minutes, turning often.

Serve and enjoy.

Nutrition: (Per serving)

Calories: 216

Net carbs: 4g

Fat: 19g

Protein: 25g

Beef and Cheese Gratin

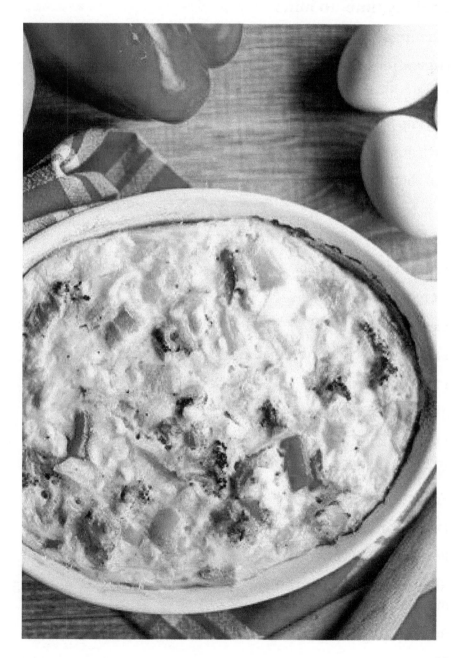

Difficulty Level: 2/5

Preparation time: 10 minutes

Cooking time: 10 mins

Servings: 4

Ingredients

1 ½ lb. steak mince

2/3 cup beef stock

3 oz. mozzarella or cheddar cheese, grated

3 oz. butter, melted

7 oz. breadcrumbs

1 tablespoon extra-virgin olive oil

1 x roast vegetable pack

1 x red onion, diced

1 x red pepper, diced

1 x 14 oz. can chopped tomatoes

1 x zucchini, diced

3 cloves garlic, crushed

1 tablespoon Worcestershire sauce

For the topping...

Fresh thyme

Directions:

Pop a skillet over a medium heat and add the oil.

Add the red pepper, onion, zucchini and garlic. Cook for 5 minutes.

Add the beef and cook for five minutes.

Throw in the tinned tomatoes, beef stock and Worcestershire sauce then stir well.

Bring to the boil then simmer for 6 minutes.

Divide between the bowl and top with the thyme.

Serve and enjoy.

Nutrition: (Per serving)

Calories: 678

Net carbs: 24g

Fat: 45g

Protein: 48g

Greek Beef and Veggie Skewers

Difficulty Level: 2/5

Preparation time: 5 minutes

Cooking time: 30 mins

Servings: 6-8

Ingredients

For the beef skewers...

1 ½ lb. skirt steak, cut into cubes

1 teaspoon grated lemon zest

½ teaspoon coriander seeds, ground

½ teaspoon salt

2 garlic cloves, chopped

2 tablespoons olive oil

2 bell peppers, seeded and cubed

4 small green zucchinis, cubed

24 cherry tomatoes

2 tablespoons extra virgin olive oil

To serve...

Store-bought hummus

1 lemon, cut into wedges

Directions:

Grab a large bowl and add all the ingredients. Stir well.

Cover and pop into the fridge for at least 30 minutes, preferably overnight.

Preheat the grill to high and oil the grate.

Take a medium bowl and add the peppers, zucchini, tomatoes and oil. Season well

Just before cooking, start threading everything onto the skewers. Alternate veggies and meat as you wish.

Pop into the grill and cook for 5 minutes on each side.

Serve and enjoy.

Nutrition: (Per serving)

Calories: 938

Net carbs: 65g

Fat: 25g

Protein: 87g

Pork Tenderloin with Orzo
Difficulty Level: 2/5

Preparation time: 10 minutes

Cooking time: 10 mins

Servings: 6

Ingredients

1-1/2 lb. pork tenderloin

1 teaspoon coarsely ground pepper

2 tablespoons extra virgin olive oil

3 quarts water

1 1/4 cups uncooked orzo pasta

1/4 teaspoon salt

6 oz. fresh baby spinach

1 cup grape tomatoes, halved

3/4 cup crumbled feta cheese

Directions:

Place the pork onto a flat surface and rub with the pepper.

Cut into the 1" cubes.

Place a skillet over a medium heat and add the oil.

Add the pork and cook for 10 minutes until no longer pink.

Fill a Dutch oven with water and place over a medium heat. Bring to a boil.

Stir in the orzo and cook uncovered for 8-10 minutes.

Stir through the spinach then drain.

Add the tomatoes to the pork, heat through then stir through orzo and cheese.

Nutrition: (Per serving)

Calories: 372

Net carbs: 34g

Fat: 11g

Protein: 31g

Moroccan Lamb Flatbreads

Difficulty Level: 2/5

Preparation time: 5 minutes

Cooking time: 25 mins

Servings: 6

Ingredients

1 ½ lb. ground lamb

1 ½ cups chopped zucchini

1 ¼ cups medium salsa

2 cups julienned carrots, divided

1/2 cup dried apricots, coarsely chopped

2 tablespoons apricot preserves

1 tablespoon grated lemon zest

1 tablespoon Moroccan seasoning (*ras el hanout*)

1/2 teaspoon garlic powder

To serve...

3 naan flat breads

1/3 cup crumbled feta cheese

2 tablespoons chopped fresh mint

Directions:

Find a large skillet and place over a medium heat.

Add the lamb and cook for 10 minutes until no longer pink, stirring and breaking up as it cooks.

Drain away any excess fat.

Add the remaining ingredients then stir and cook for 7-10 minutes.

Place the naan onto plates, spoon over the lamb mixture then top with the feta and mint.

Cut into wedges then serve and enjoy.

Nutrition: (Per serving)

Calories: 423

Net carbs: 15g

Fat: 19g

Protein: 24g

Greek Lamb Burgers

Difficulty Level: 2/5

Preparation time: 5 minutes

Cooking time: 30 mins

Servings: 8

Ingredients

2 lb. ground lamb

1 small red onion, grated

2 garlic cloves, minced

1 cup chopped fresh parsley

10 mint leaves, chopped

2 ½ teaspoons dry oregano

2 teaspoons ground cumin

½ teaspoon paprika

½ teaspoon cayenne pepper, optional

Salt and pepper, to taste

Extra virgin olive oil

To serve...

Greek pita bread or buns

Tzatziki sauce

Sliced tomatoes

Sliced green bell pepper

Sliced cucumbers

Sliced red onions

Pitted Kalamata olives, sliced

Crumbled feta

Directions:

Preheat your outdoor grill on medium whilst you prepare your burgers.

Grab a large mixing bowl and add the lamb, onions, garlic, herbs, oregano, cumin, paprika and cayenne.

Season well, drizzle with olive oil and mix everything together using your hands.

Shape into 8 balls then press into patties. Use your thumb to make a small depression into the middle of each.

Oil the grill and place the burger patties on top.

Cook for 5-10 minutes until cooked, turning halfway through.

Leave to rest for 5-10 minutes then serve and enjoy.

Nutrition: (Per serving)

Calories: 77

Net carbs: 6g

Fat: 5g

Protein: 3g

Broiled Swordfish with Oven-Roasted Tomato Sauce

Difficulty Level: 3/5

Preparation time: 5 minutes

Cooking time: 25 mins

Servings: 4

Ingredients

4 x 4 oz. fresh or frozen swordfish steaks, cut about 1" thick

Extra virgin olive oil

1 lb. Roma tomatoes, cored and quartered

½ small onion, peeled and quartered

3 cloves garlic, peeled

¼ teaspoon salt

¼ teaspoon crushed red pepper

2 tablespoons tomato paste

1 teaspoon snipped fresh rosemary

½ cup vegetable broth

2 tablespoons heavy cream

1 tablespoon olive oil

½ teaspoon freshly ground black pepper

2 tablespoons finely snipped fresh basil or Italian parsley

Directions:

Preheat the broiler and lightly grease a 15 x 10" baking pan with olive oil.

Place the tomatoes, onion and garlic into the pan and then season well.

Broil for 10 minutes.

Add the tomato paste and stir well to coat.

Broil for 5 more minutes.

Place the tomatoes into your food processor with the rosemary then cover and blend until smooth.

Pour into a saucepan and stir through the broth. Bring to a boil, stirring often.

Reduce the heat then cook for 15 minutes.

Add the heavy cream then stir through. Cover with the lid and keep warm.

Cover a broiler pan with foil.

Next season both sides of the fish with oil, season well with pepper and place onto the broiler pan.

Broil for 10-12 minutes until cooked.

Serve the fish with the sauce then enjoy!

Nutrition: (Per serving)

Calories: 254

Net carbs: 7g

Fat: 12g

Protein: 24g

Pan-Seared Citrus Shrimp
Difficulty Level: 2/5

Preparation time: 10 minutes

Cooking time: 15 mins

Servings: 4

Ingredients

1 tablespoon olive oil

Juice of 2 oranges

Juice of 3 lemons

5 garlic cloves, minced or pressed

1 tablespoon finely chopped red onion or shallot

1 tablespoon chopped fresh parsley

Pinch red pepper flakes

Salt and pepper, to taste

3 lb. medium shrimp peeled and deveined

1 medium orange, cut into wedges or slices

1 medium lemon, cut into wedges

Method

Find a medium bowl and add the olive oil, orange juice, lemon juice, garlic, onion, 2 teaspoons of the parsley and a pinch of red pepper flakes. Stir well to combine.

Pour the mixture into a large skillet and place over a medium heat.

Bring to a simmer and cook for 5-8 minutes until reduced to half.

Add the shrimp, season well then cover and cook for about 5 minutes until no longer pink.

Top with the rest of the parsley and with the lemon and orange slices, then serve and enjoy.

Nutrition: (Per serving)

Calories: 262

Net carbs: 18g

Fat: 6g

Protein: 38g

Quinoa and Halibut Bowl

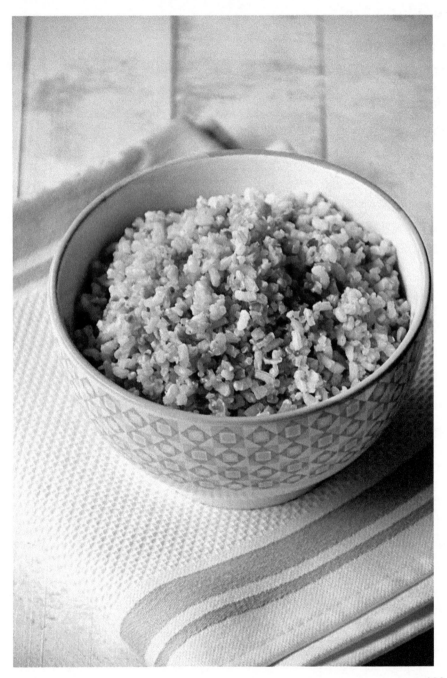

Difficulty Level: 2/5

Preparation time: 5 minutes

Cooking time: 20 mins

Servings: 4

Ingredients

2 tablespoons extra virgin olive oil

2 teaspoons ground cumin

1 teaspoon dried rosemary

1 tablespoon ground coriander

2 teaspoons dried oregano

2 teaspoons ground cinnamon

1 teaspoon salt

For the bowl...

2 cups cooked quinoa

1 avocado, sliced

1 cup cherry tomatoes, cut in half

1/2 cup pitted kalamata olives, sliced

1 cucumber, cubed cucumber

Greek dressing

1 lemon

Directions:

Preheat your oven to 435°F.

Find a small bowl and add the cumin, rosemary, coriander, oregano, cinnamon and salt. Stir well.

Place the halibut onto a flat surface and rub with the spice mix.

Find a skillet, add enough olive oil to cover the bottom and then sear the halibut.

Once brown, pop into the oven and cook for about 5 minutes.

Meanwhile, place the quinoa, salad ingredients into the bowl and drizzle with the dressing.

Remove the fish from the oven then place it on top of the quinoa.

Serve and enjoy.

Nutrition: (Per serving)

Calories: 608

Net carbs: 75g

Fat: 29g

Protein: 16g

Barramundi in Parchment with Lemons, Dates and Toasted Almonds
Difficulty Level: 2/5

Preparation time: 5 minutes

Cooking time: 22 mins

Servings: 2

Ingredients

2 x 6 oz. barramundi fillets

1 whole lemon

1 medium shallot, peeled and thinly sliced

6 oz. baby spinach

2 tablespoons extra virgin olive oil

1/4 cup unsalted almonds, coarsely chopped

4 Medjool dates, pitted and finely chopped

1/4 cup fresh flat-leaf parsley, chopped

Salt and pepper, to taste

Directions:

Preheat the oven to 400°F.

Season the barramundi with salt and pepper then pop to one side.

Remove the zest from the entire lemon then cut half of the lemon into 4-5 slices and juice the other half.

Place two 12 x 12" piece of baking parchment side by side and put half of the shallots and half of the spinach into each. Season well.

Place the barramundi on top, add the lemon slices and drizzle with olive oil.

Close the parchment paper by folding then place both packages onto a baking sheet.

Pop into the oven for 10-12 minutes.

Meanwhile, place a small skillet over a medium heat and add a small amount of oil.

Add the chopped almonds and sauté for 2 minutes.

Add the dates and cook for a further 2 minutes until warmed through.

Remove from the heat then add the lemon zest, lemon juice and parsley.

Season well then serve and enjoy.

Nutrition: (Per serving)

Calories: 477

Net carbs: 45g

Fat: 25g

Protein: 24g

Sardine Fish Cakes
Difficulty Level: 2/5

Preparation time: 5 minutes

Cooking time: 20 mins

Servings: 6

Ingredients

6 fresh cleaned sardines

2 garlic cloves, minced

1 medium onion, finely chopped

2 tablespoons fresh dill, chopped

1 cup breadcrumbs

1 free-range egg

2 tablespoons lemon juice

Pinch of salt & pepper, to taste

5 tablespoons extra virgin olive oil

Wedges of lemon, to serve

Directions:

Find a medium bowl and add the sardines, mashing well with a fork.

Add the remaining ingredients (except the olive oil and lemon) and stir well to combine.

Shape into six cakes.

Place a skillet over a medium heat and add the oil.

Fry the cakes for a few minutes each side until brown then serve and enjoy.

Nutrition: (Per serving)

Calories: 197

Net carbs: 9g

Fat: 14g

Protein: 8g

Baked Salmon Tacos

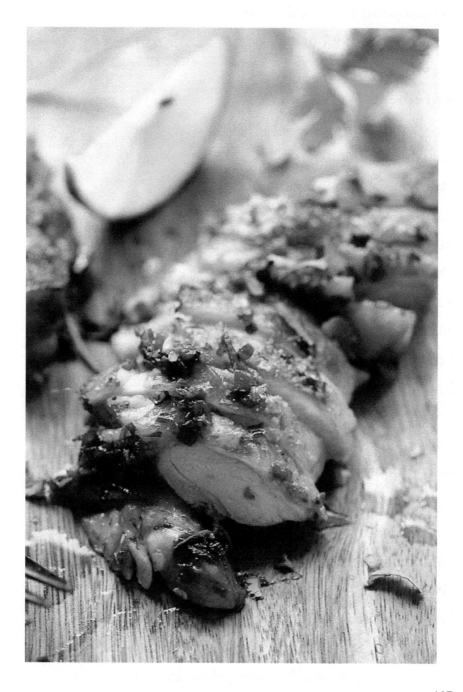

Difficulty Level: 2/5

Preparation time: 5 minutes

Cooking time: 25 mins

Servings: 8

Ingredients

8-10 corn tortillas

½ lb. fresh salmon

1 teaspoon olive oil

Garlic powder, to taste

Ground cumin, to taste

Chili powder (optional), to taste

Salt & pepper, to taste

For the sauce...

1 cup plain Greek yogurt

Juice of 1/2 lime

1 clove garlic, minced

Handful fresh cilantro, chopped

For the toppings...

1 avocado, diced

Shredded iceberg lettuce, to taste

Lime wedges, to taste

Directions:

Preheat your oven to 375°F and line a baking sheet with foil.

Wrap the tortillas in foil and place into the oven.

Place the salmon onto the baking sheet and drizzle with oil.

Sprinkle with garlic, cumin, chili and salt and pepper.

Pop into the oven for 10 minutes until cooked through.

Meanwhile, find a medium bowl and add the ingredients for the sauce. Stir well then pop to one side.

When the salmon is cooked, remove from the oven and cut into bite-sized pieces.

Remove the tortillas from the oven and fill with the salmon, toppings and sauce.

Serve and enjoy.

Nutrition: (Per serving)

Calories: 92

Net carbs: 13g

Fat: 2g

Protein: 7g

Lightning Source UK Ltd.
Milton Keynes UK
UKHW020657310521
384668UK00001B/85